Gluten Free is NOT Fun for Me!

Written and illustrated by

Kimberly Shaw

PAGE PUBLISHING, INC.
Conneaut Lake, PA

First originally published by Page Publishing 2020

ISBN 978-1-6624-0431-3 (pbk)
ISBN 978-1-6624-0432-0 (digital)

Printed in the United States of America

This book is dedicated to my daughter Daysha, my love Phil, my sister Page, and my amazing friends for always supporting and standing by me.

Gluten-free is not fun for me,
It is an autoimmune disorder that I have called **celiac disease**.

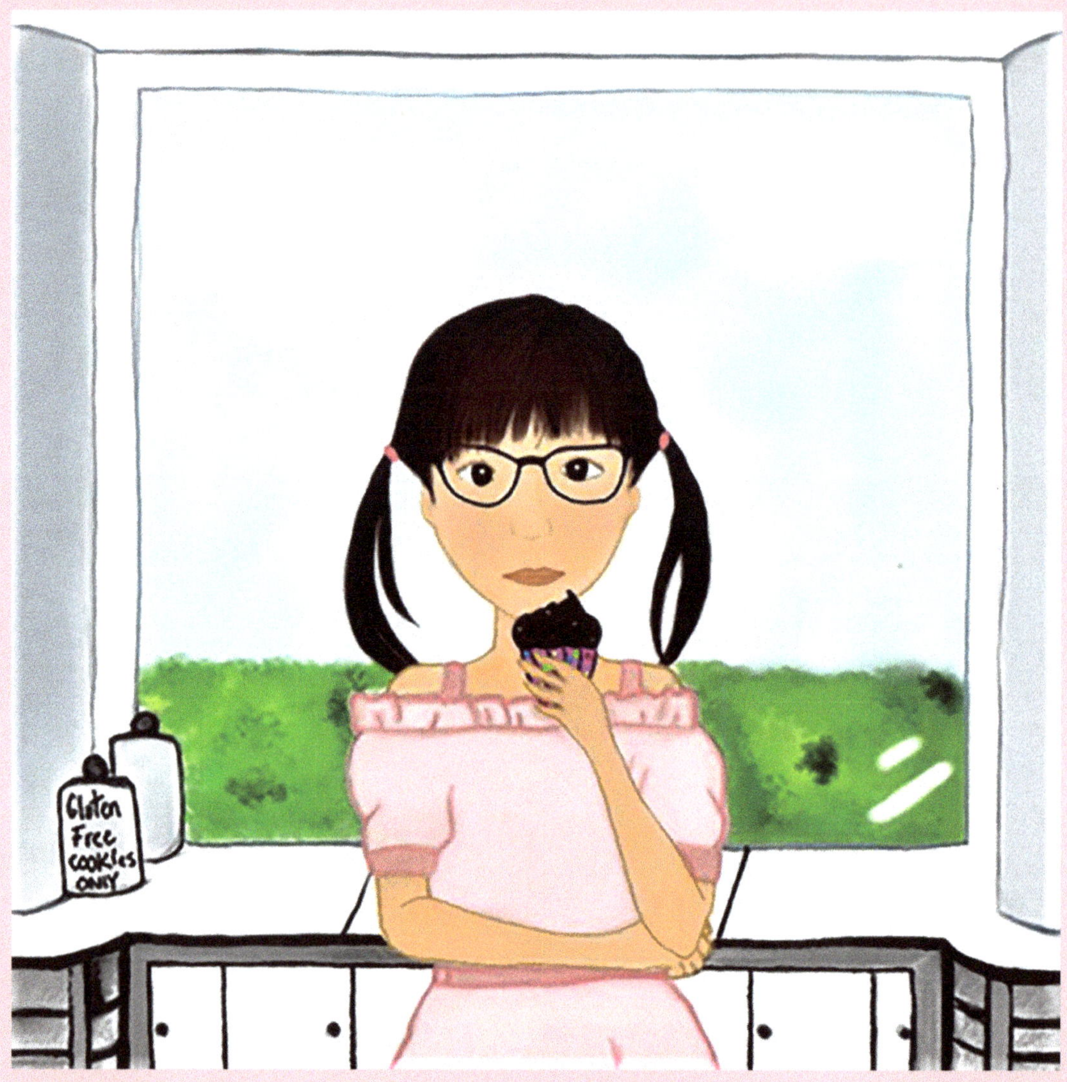

But before you *panic!*
I want you to know you can't catch *celiac*' it's not a *flu* or *cold*.

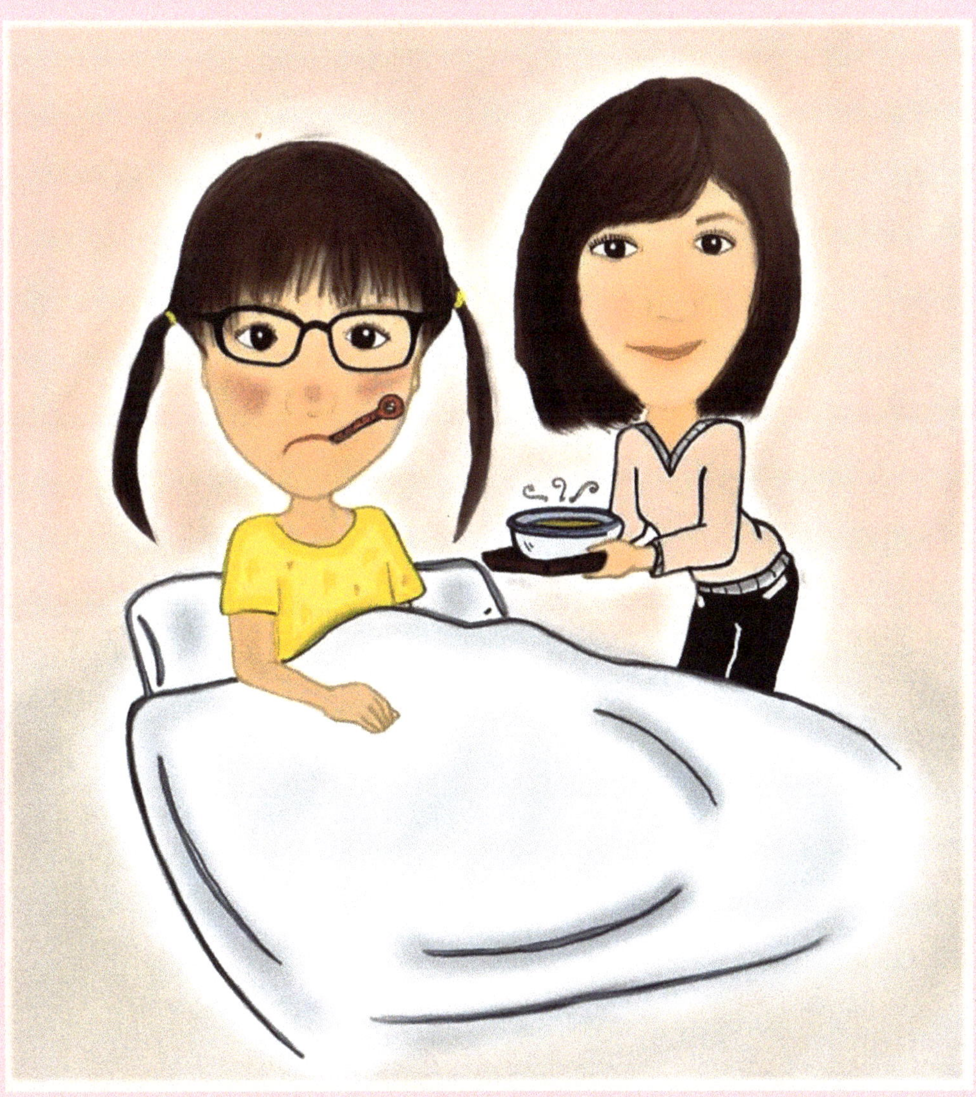

And what I'm about to tell you may sound a little crazy…

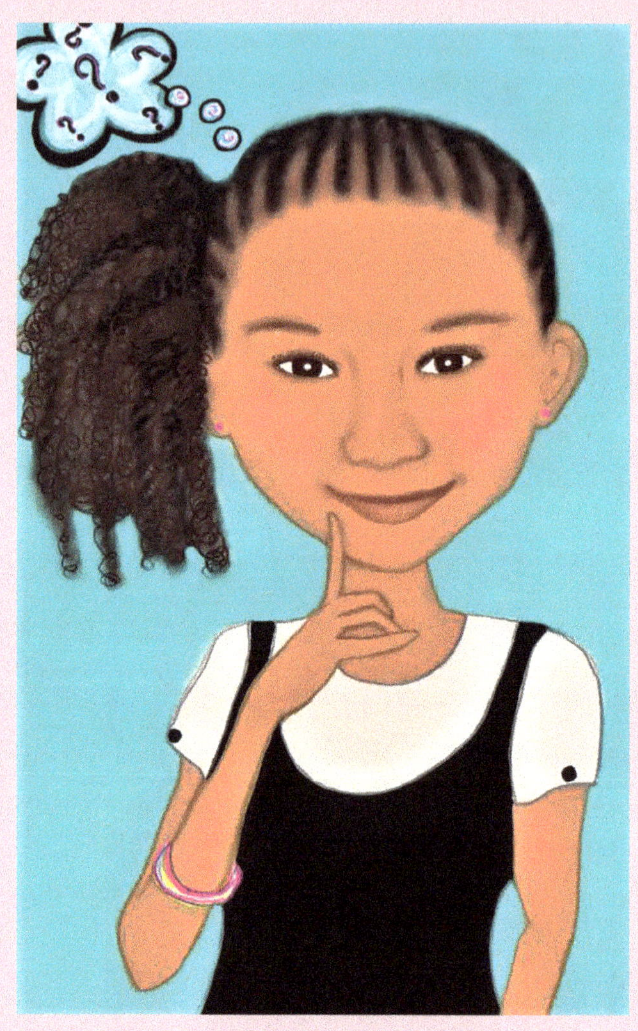

But what may be good for you is not always good for me! Because celiac is **NOT** an allergy or intolerance, and there is no cure.

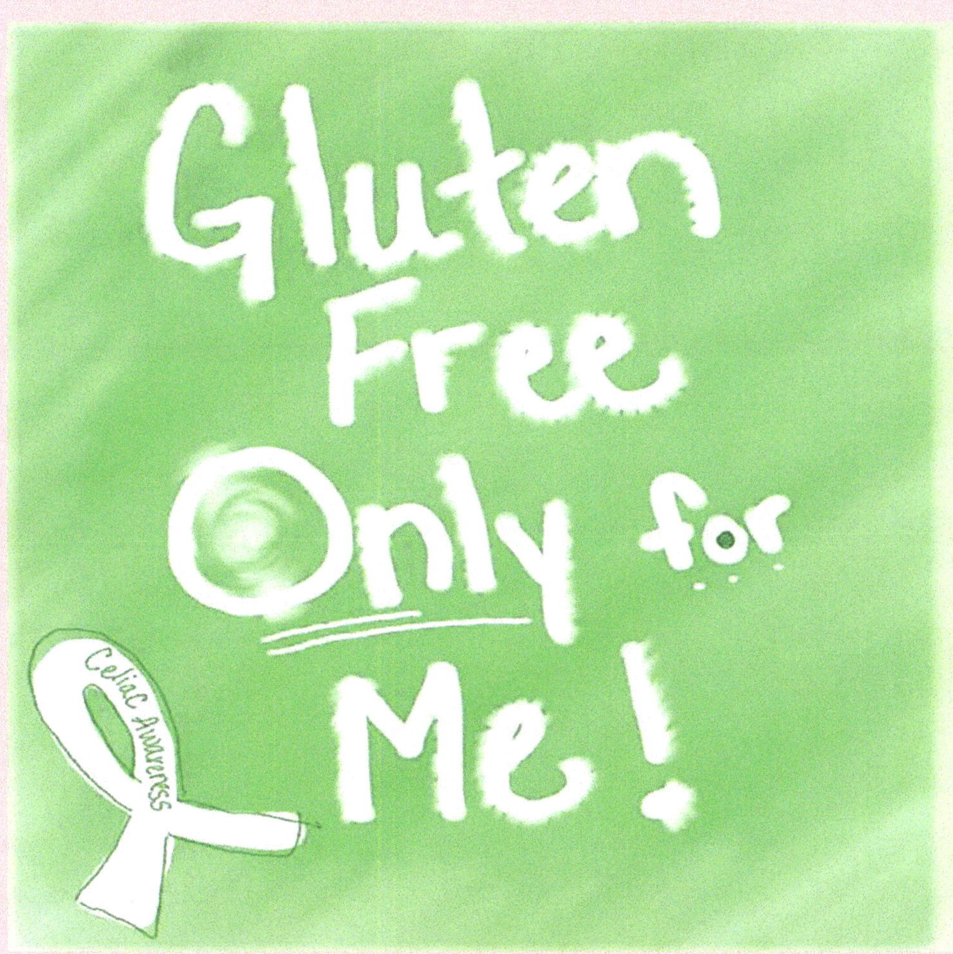

This may seem confusing at the moment, and hopefully, I can help you understand why a **gluten-free** diet is not only the **safest** but a **need**!

And no, there is no other option that is good for me!

"Gluten?" you ask, "What is that?"

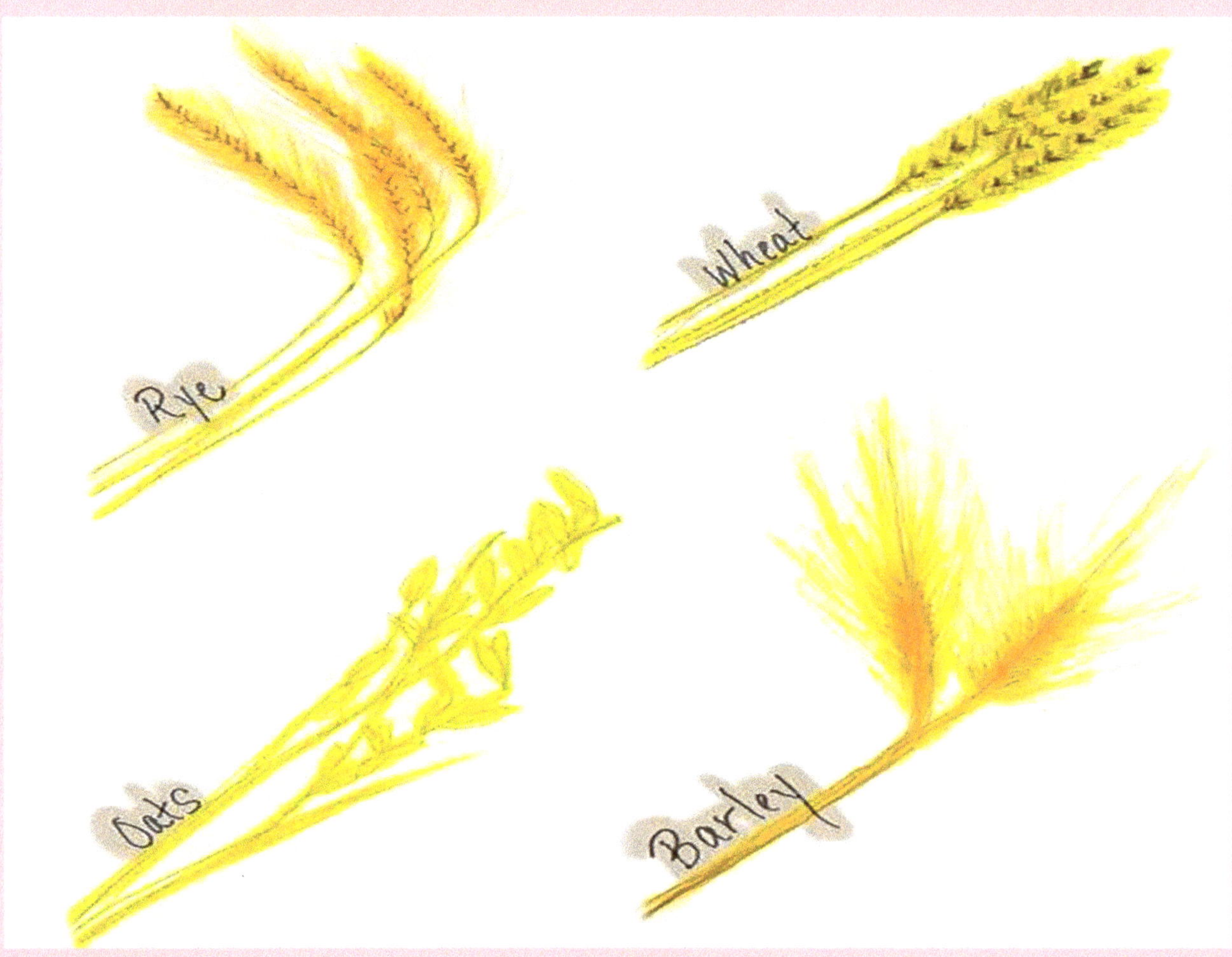

It is in wheat, oats, barley, and rye, A little ingredient that is mixed in with many different things!

It is in;
Cupcakes, Pizza, Cookies, Oatmeal and Bread!

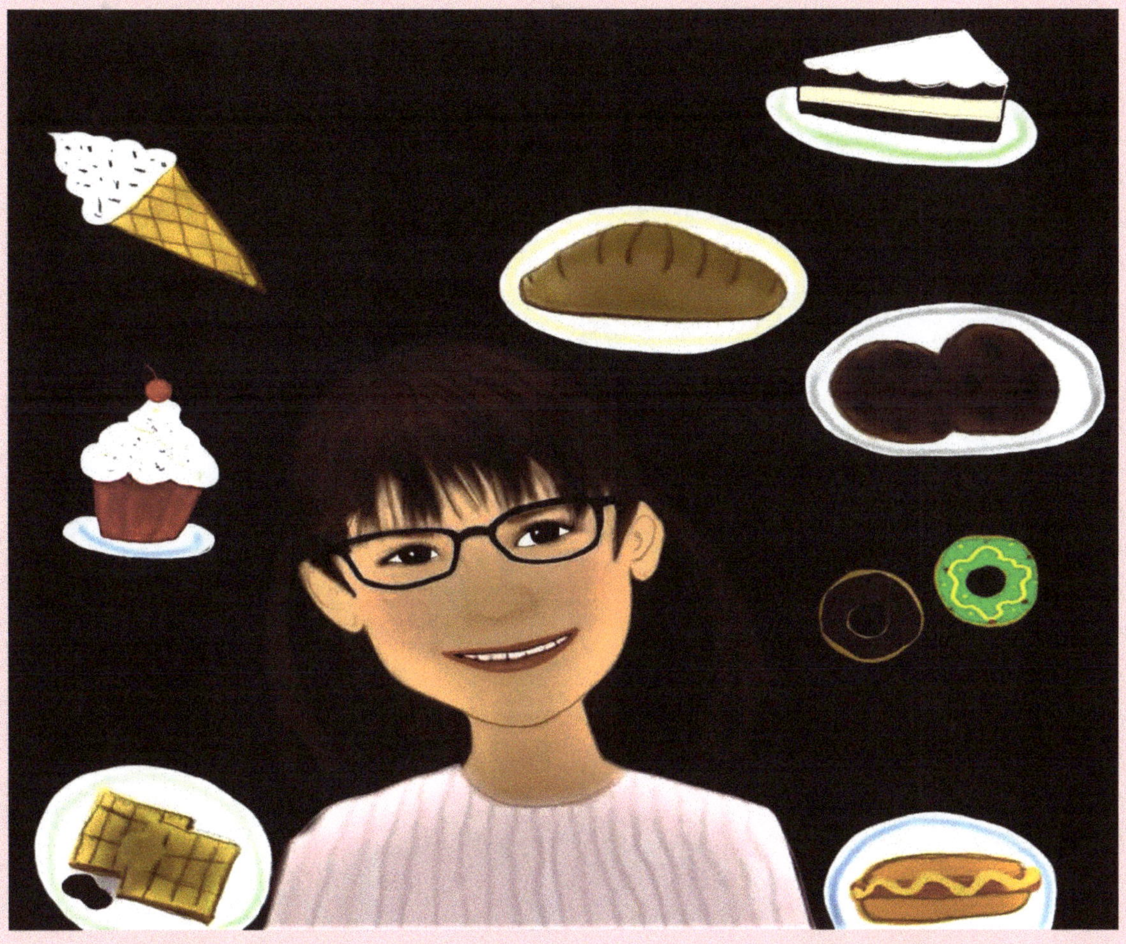

It's just not food; it's on many other items and things…
It is on **dishes, toasters, door handles, counter,** and **tabletops.**

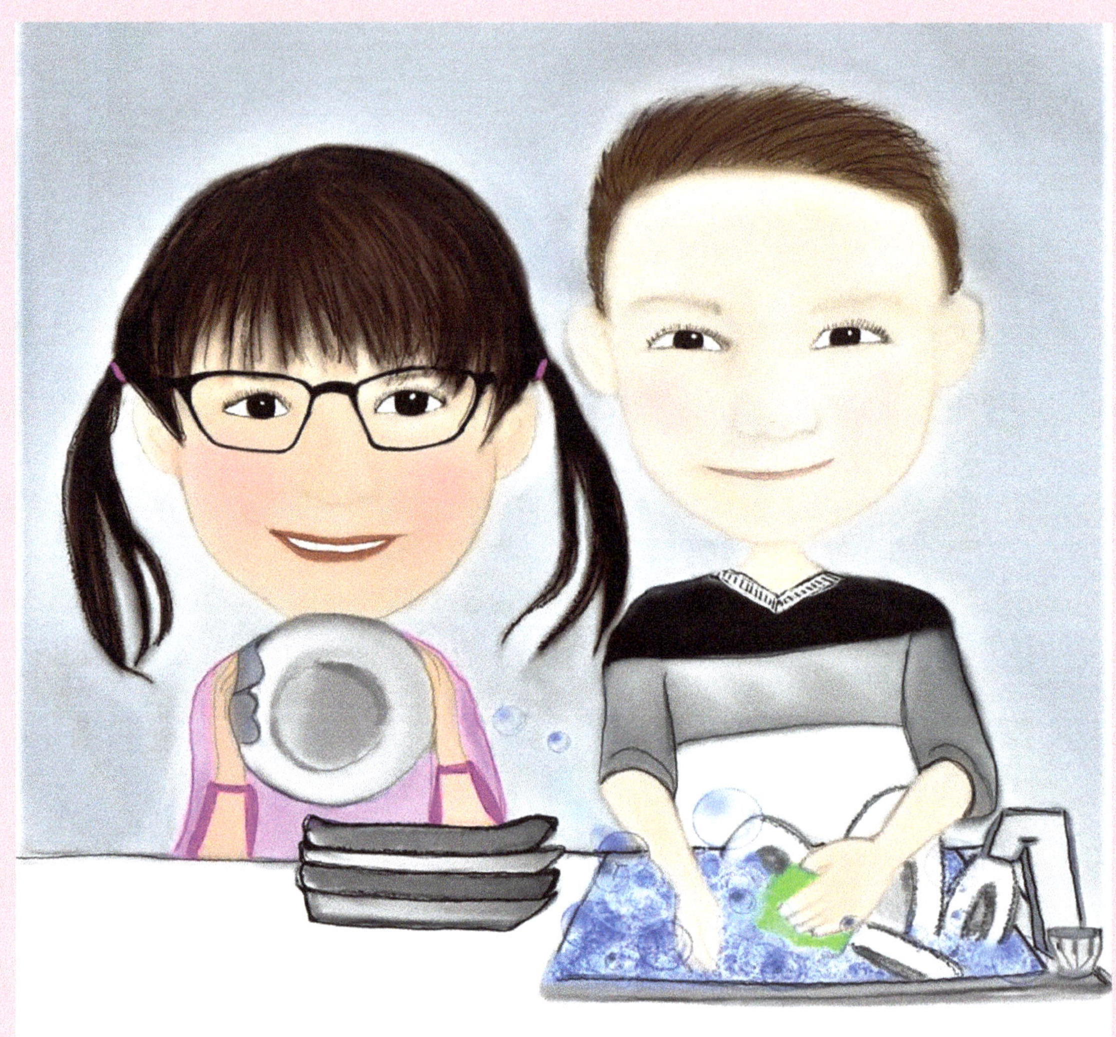

It is in **playdough, shampoo, toothpaste,** and also in the **AIR** too!

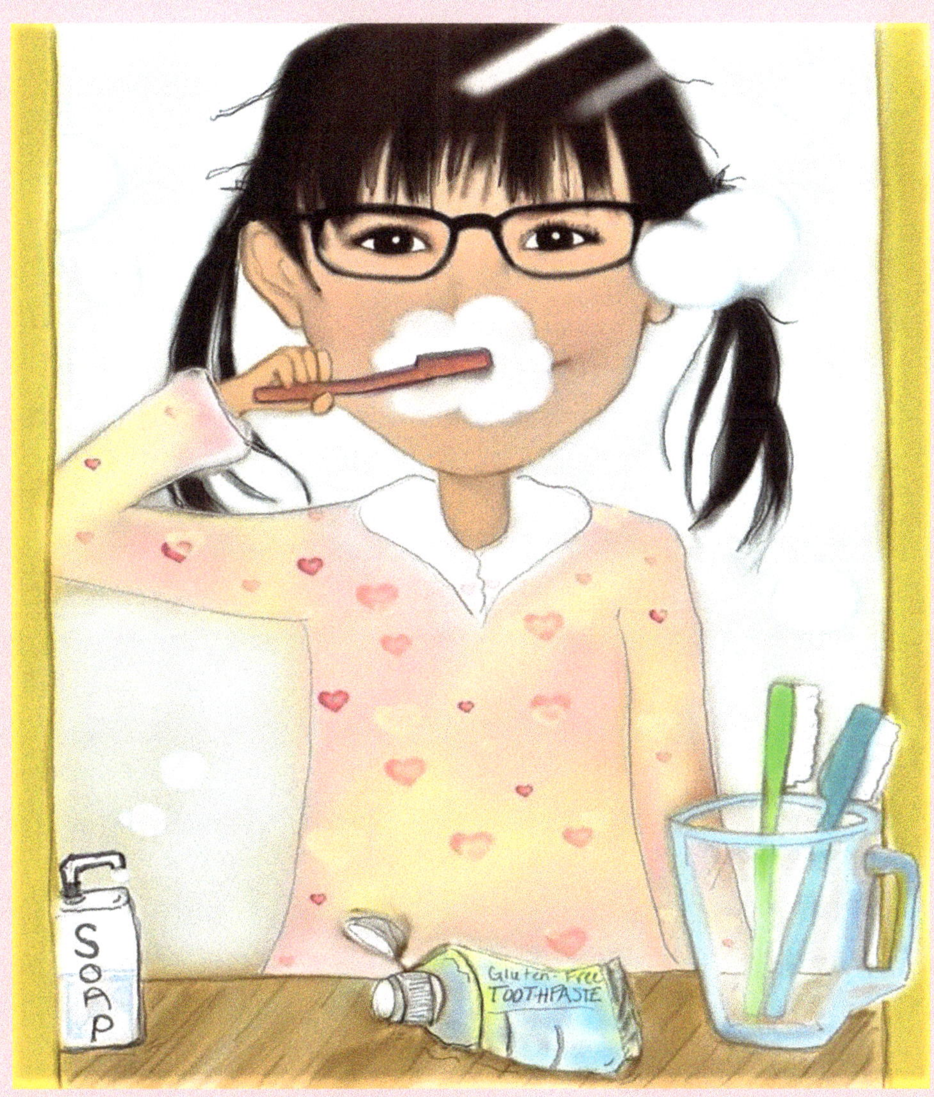

That is just naming a few.

I could list you more than one hundred items if you wanted me to.

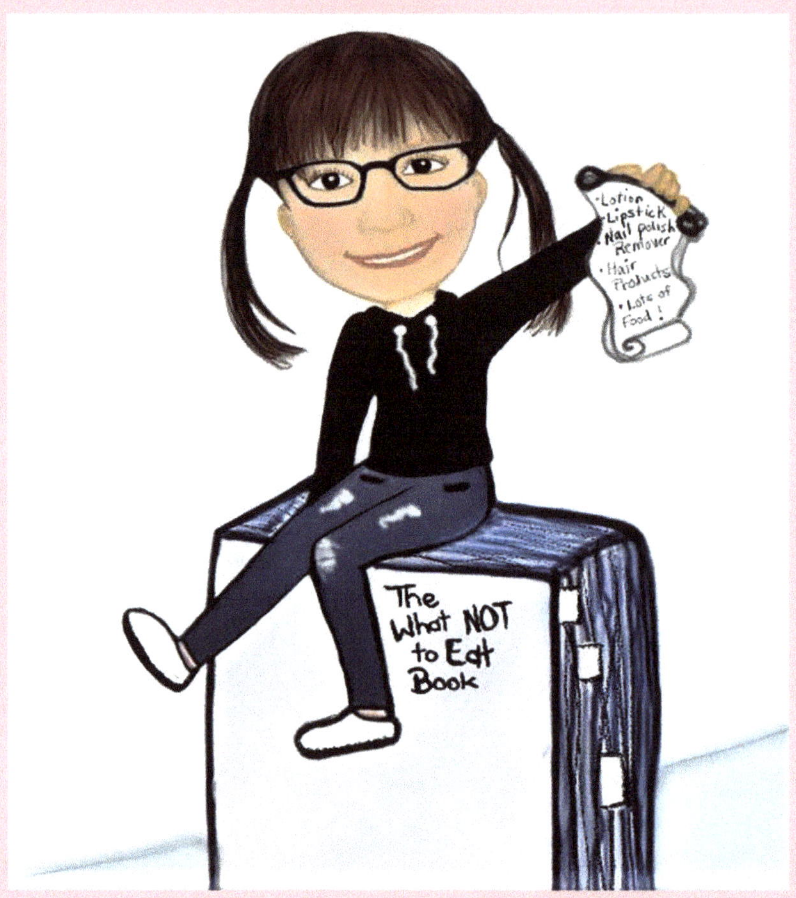

Sometimes it can be scary because it is truly everywhere!
Sad but true—if I eat gluten,
something simple as a crumb, a tiny pebble size…

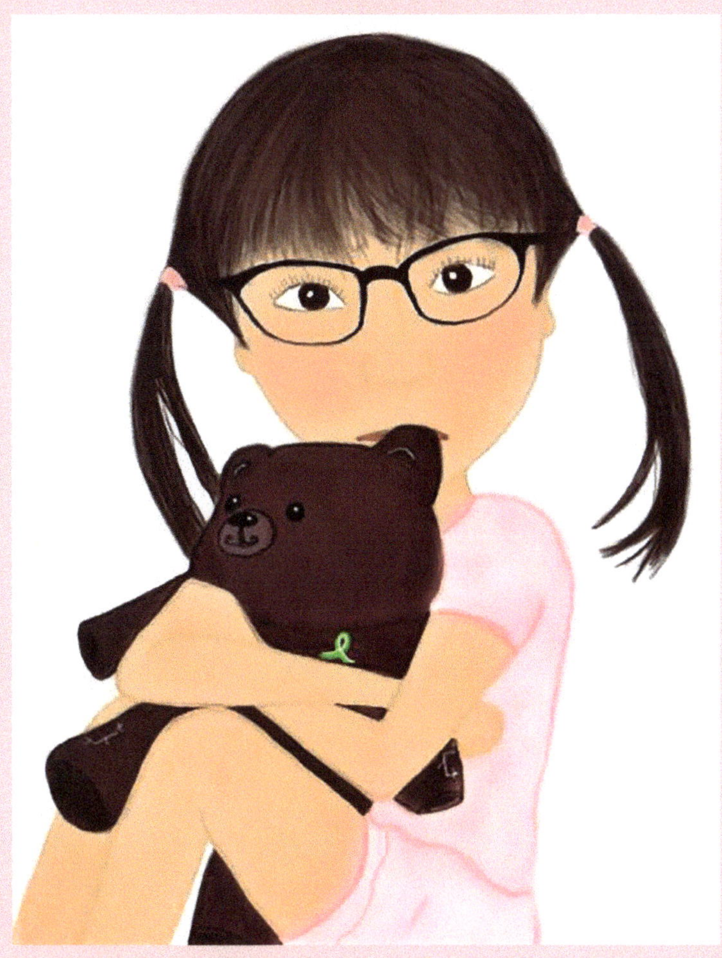

If I touch it and even breathing it in can make me feel super ill.
And there is no such thing as a cheat day!

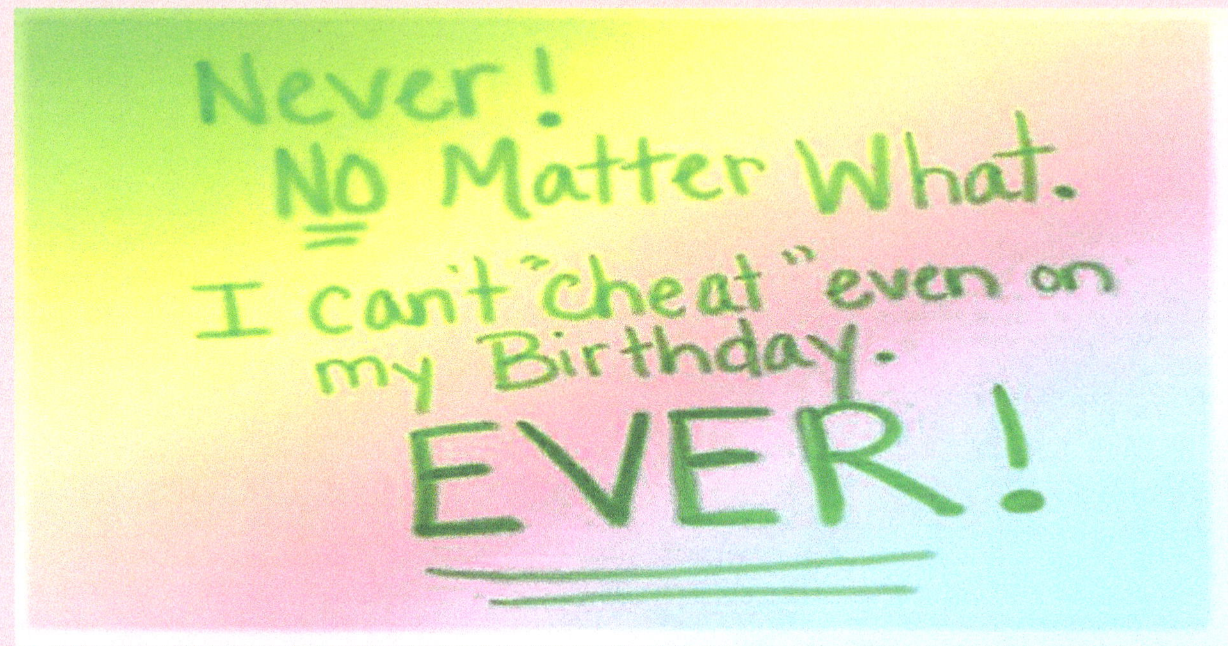

Absolutely
        NO WAY!

My belly will do more than just hurt; gluten will cause me all sorts of aches and pains.

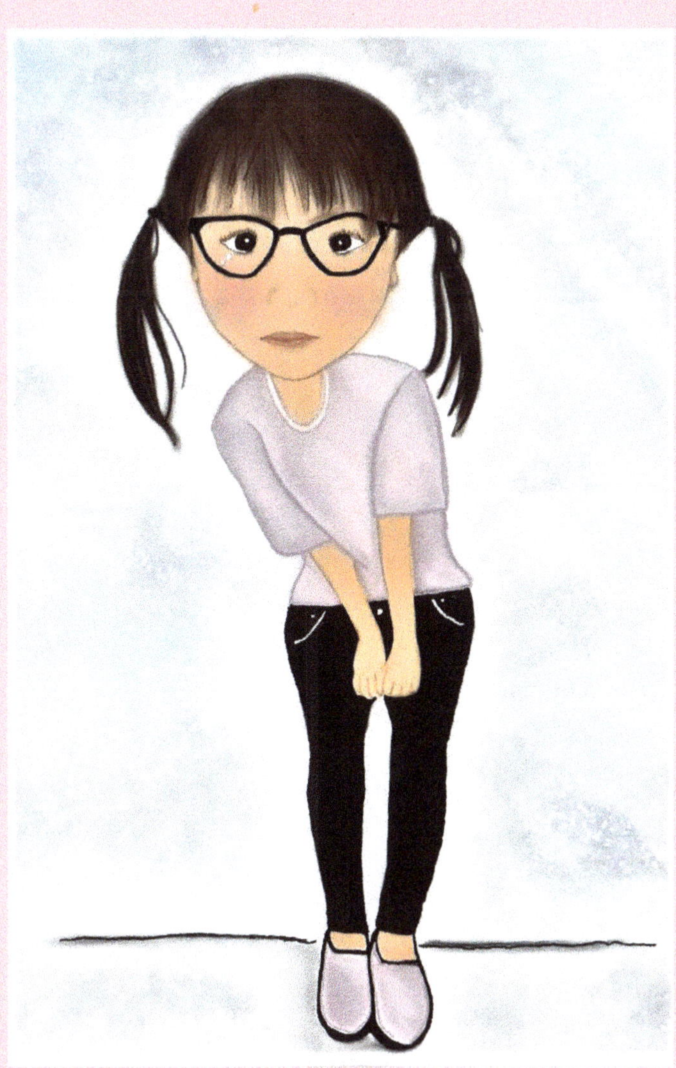

I will feel a lot of different icky things, and staying in bed all day is really no fun!

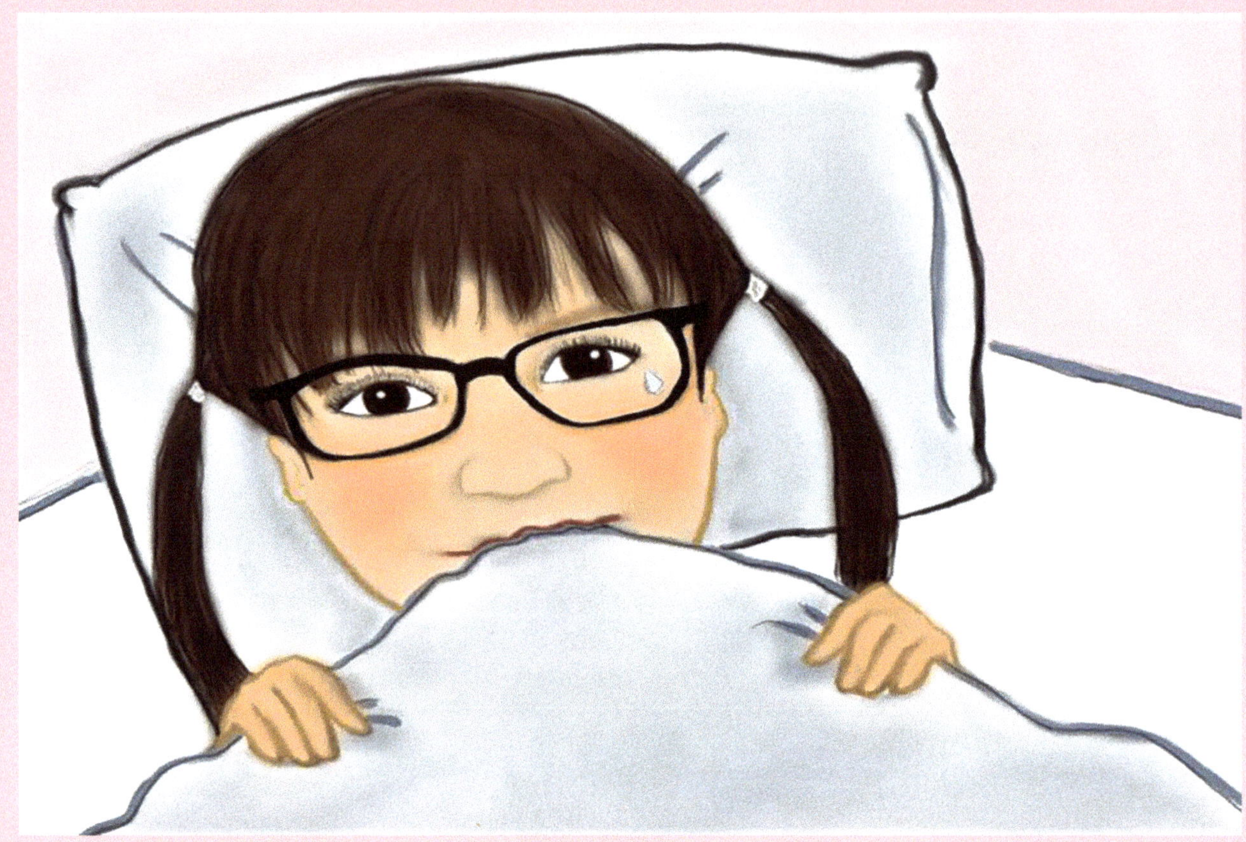

(And I have to be really careful…)
Because if I'm not, I will have to go to the hospital!

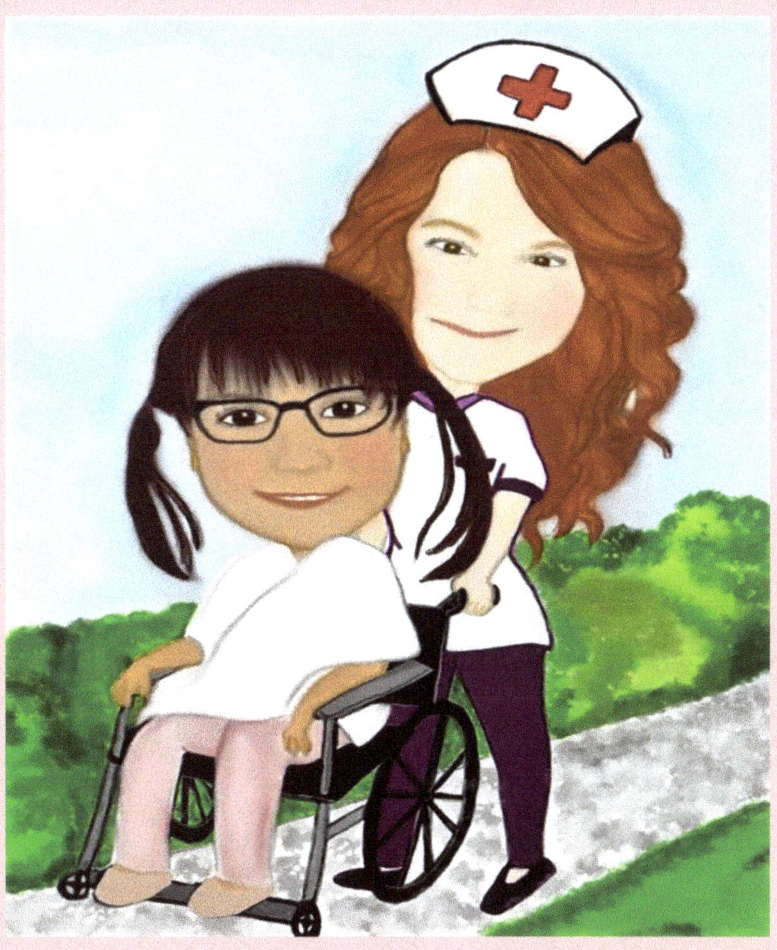

And between us,
the food is really gross there…
I'm not able to take anything to make me feel better, so all I can
do is be **STRONG.**

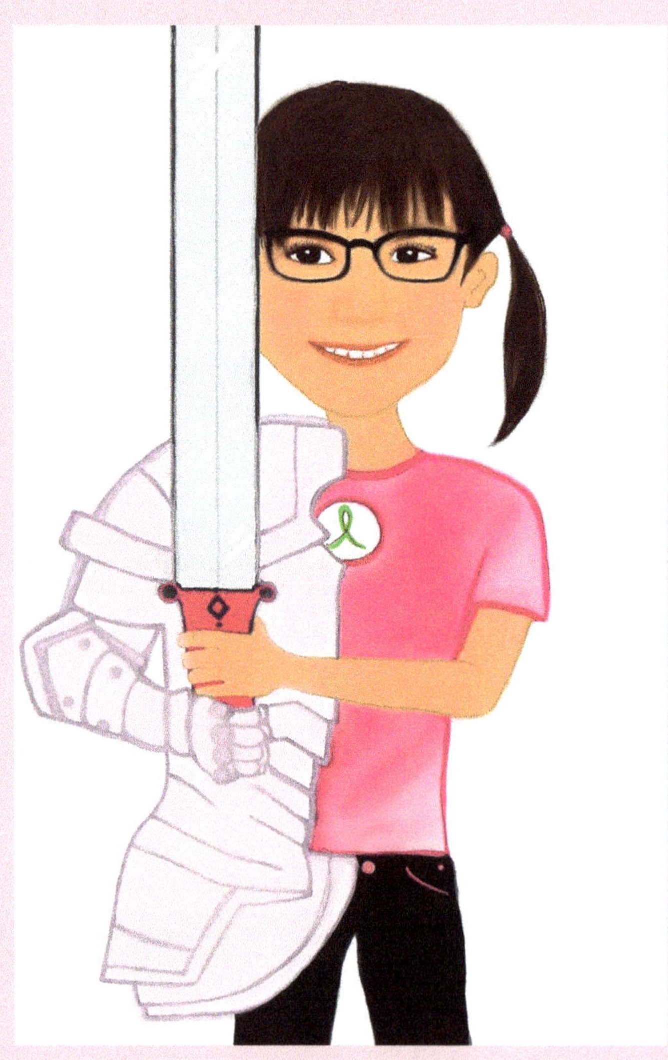

If I'm glutened by mistake because of all the crazy things that I go thorough,

The only way I can start to feel a little better is by drinking lots of water!

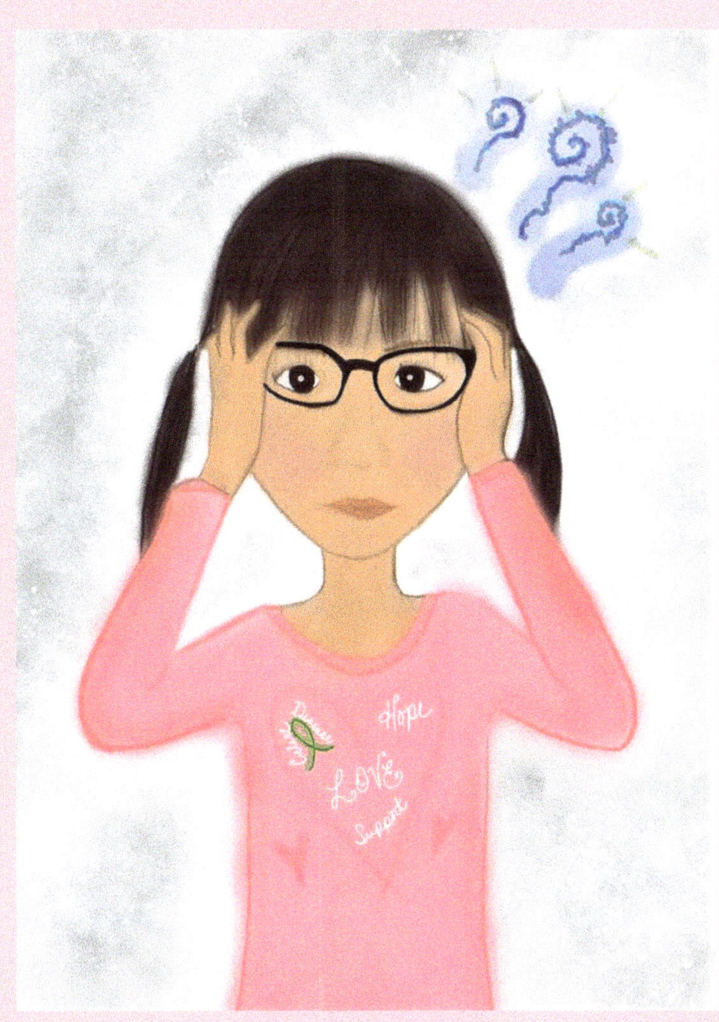

And for my breakfast, lunch, and dinner, I typically have broth.
But once my belly starts to feel a bit better,
I'm able to try gelatin, popsicles, and gluten-free toast.

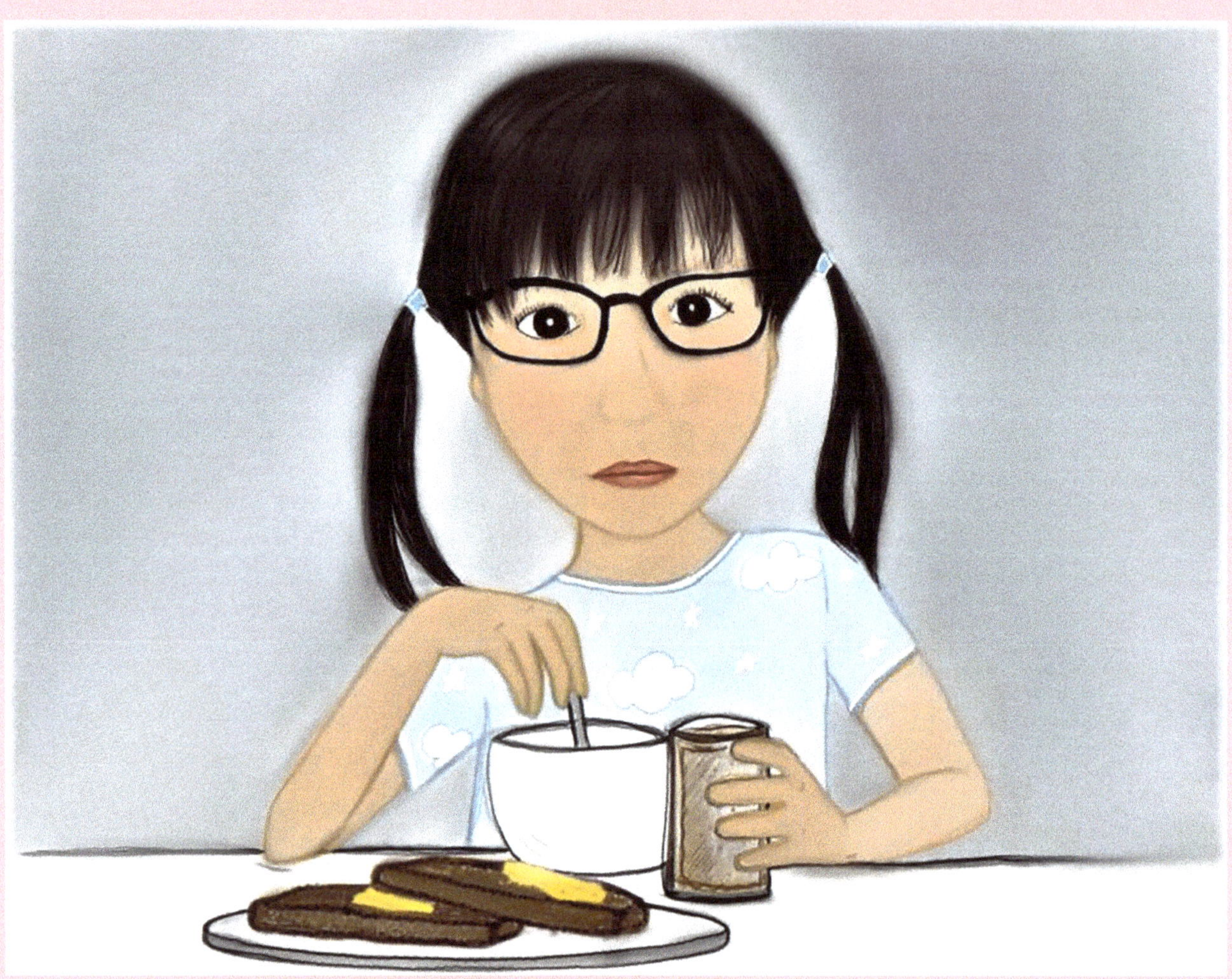

But with that said…

Celiac isn't who I am. It is my disease; it doesn't change who I will be!

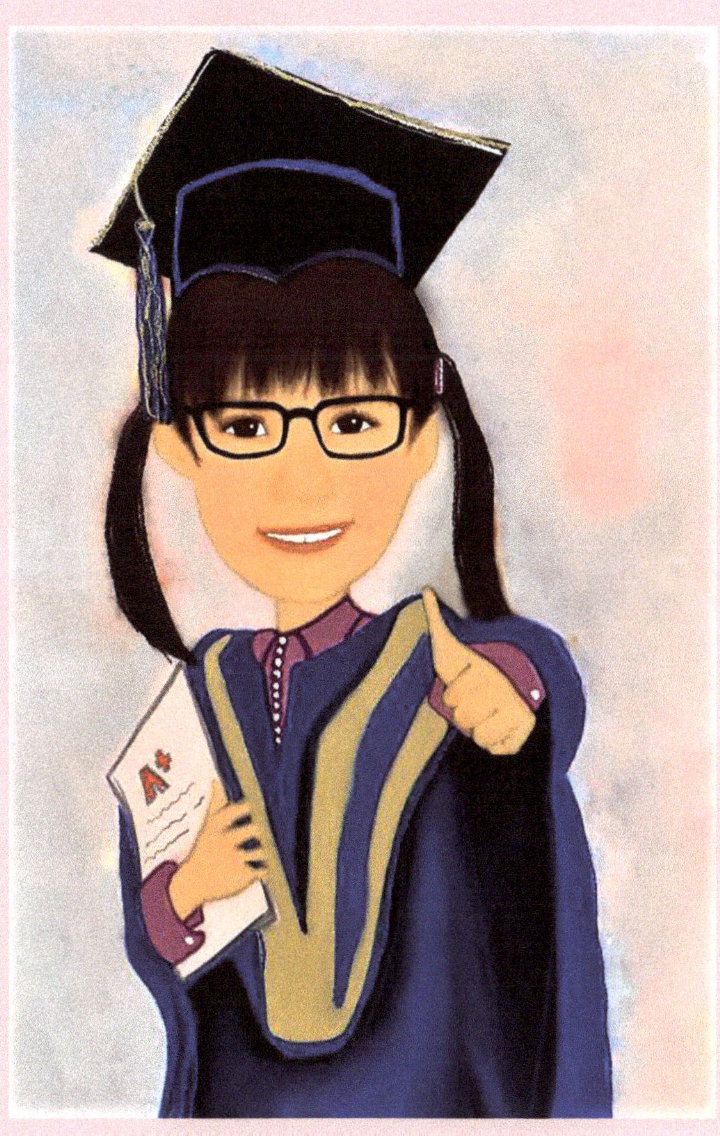

And even though I may be a **little** *different*,
I still know how to have a lot of **FUN!**

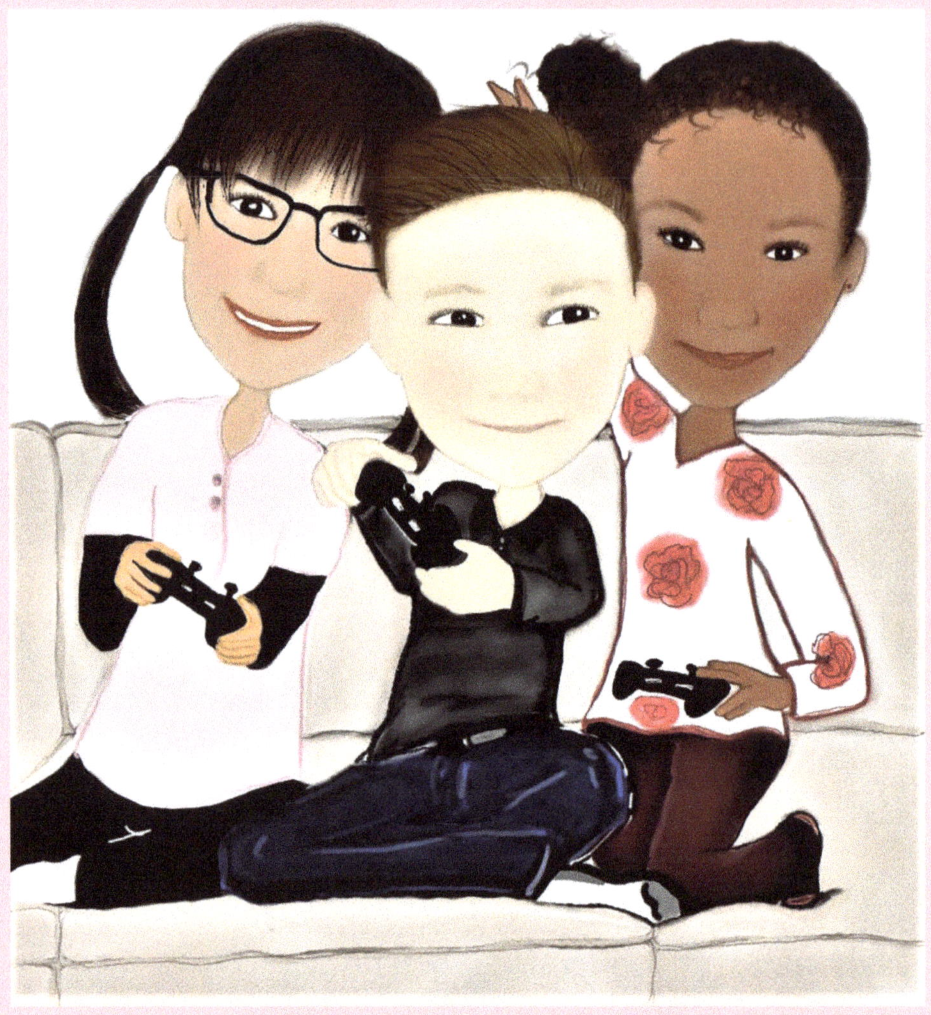

And just so you know,

I won't be sad if I can't have what you have because I have different options that are just for me.

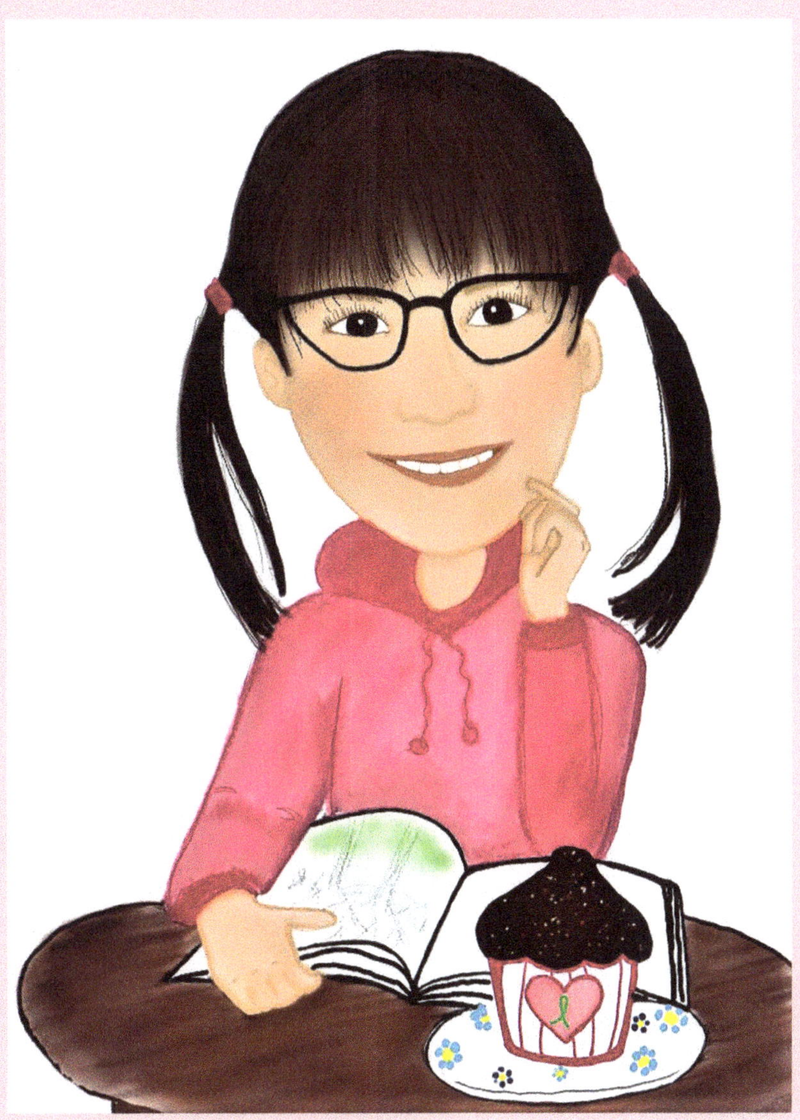

Plus, my mom always says, "Our life is like a picnic" because we bring our own food wherever we go.

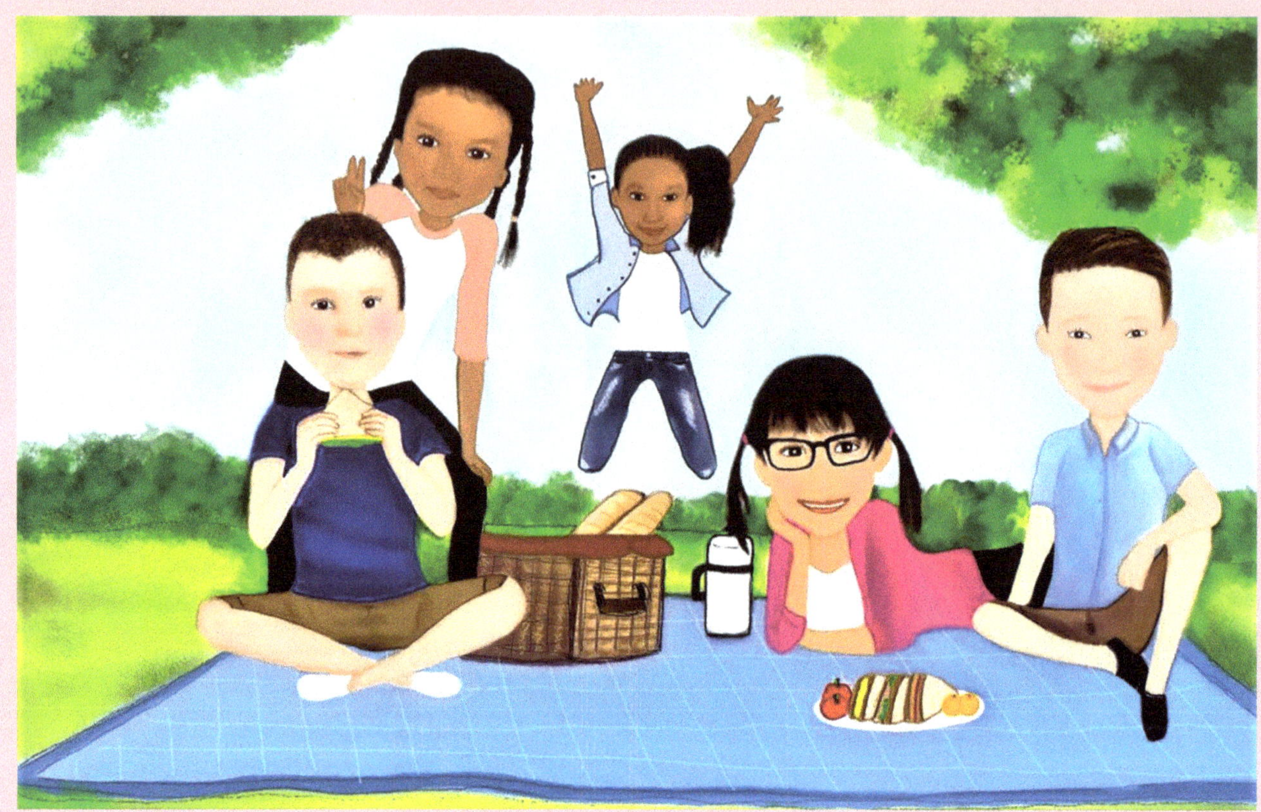

And…
we'd rather be safe than
sorry, and that is cool with me!
So now that you know a bit about celiac disease,
Please don't be upset when I cannot accept a treat.

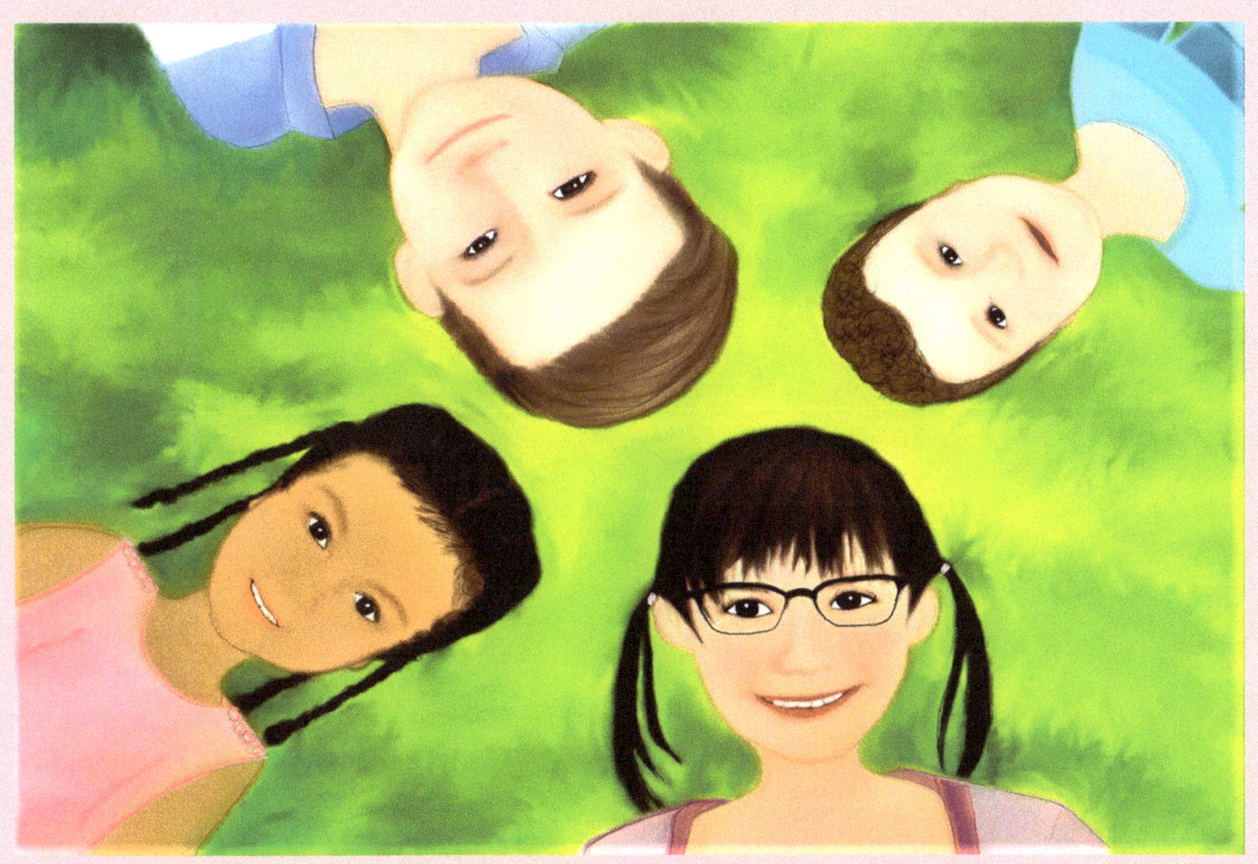

But thank you so much for taking the time to think of me!
I do ask, though, that you
Please keep your hands clean,

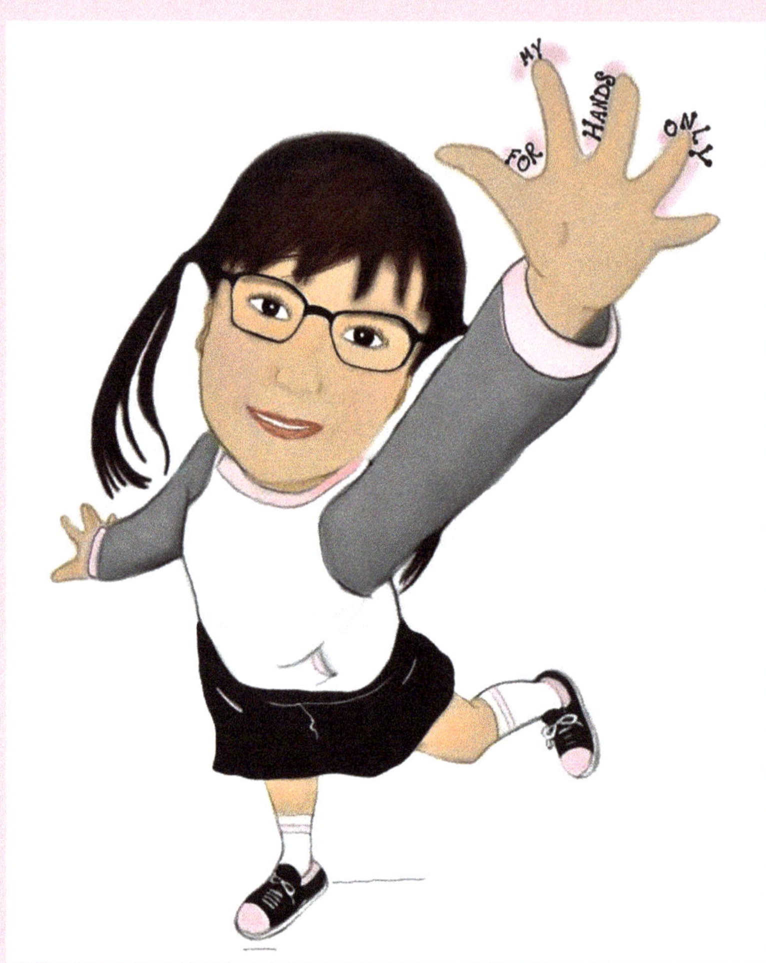

And it is SUPER DUPER important that you know…
My food *can* **ONLY** *be* **TOUCHED** *by me*!
But if in doubt, don't be scared,
you can ask me or my family anything!
We like answering your questions because awareness is something
we are really good at.

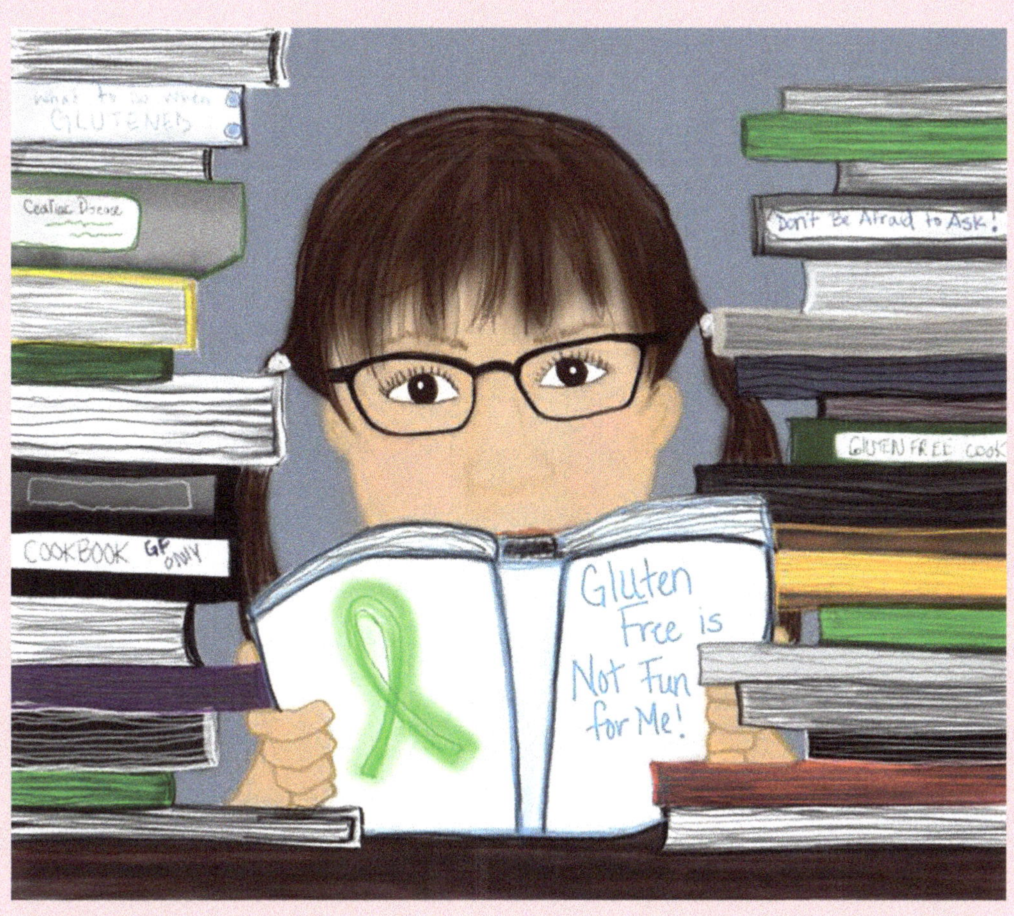

About the Author

Kim is a mom, wife, sister, aunt, best friend, and teacher. Writing and teaching have always been a passion to her, and when her and her daughter were diagnosed with celiac disease, it changed not only their lives but everyone's who was a part of their lives. When they were both diagnosed, the only information they had was a diagnosis, a "what not to eat" list (that was not informal at all); and on a whim, after googling two words "celiac disease," a website (Celiac.org) came up, and finally, she found hope. Now after seven years, a long road of health and medical conditions, learning, teaching, advocating, but mostly because of the inspiration from her daughter Daysha—whom this book is written about—her husband, Phil, sister Page, and friends, she is able to finally make her dreams come true and hopefully continue to spread awareness for those who have celiac disease or knows someone with celiac.